Let Her Go Before Death

Navigating The Breast Cancer Journey

By: Somtoochukwu Justin

Copyright

Let her go before death

Contents

AUTHORS NOTE

As the author of this comprehensive exploration into the world of breast cancer, I find myself reflecting on the profound and deeply personal nature of this subject. Breast cancer is not just a medical issue; it is a tapestry of individual stories, resilience, and hope. In this Author's Note, I want to share my personal reflections and connection to the subject that inspired me to create this work.

I, like many, have been touched by breast cancer in various ways. Whether through the experiences of friends, family members, or acquaintances, the impact of this diagnosis has been undeniable. These personal connections have driven me to understand, empathize, and contribute to the collective knowledge that empowers individuals facing the challenges of breast cancer.

My motivation for writing this book stems from a strong belief in the power of knowledge. In the face of a breast cancer diagnosis, information can be a beacon of empowerment. By providing a comprehensive guide that covers everything from the intricacies of the disease to the importance of emotional well-being, my aim is to offer a source of support and guidance for those navigating this difficult journey.

It is essential to recognize the human element at the heart of every word in this book. Each sentence is crafted with the understanding that behind every statistic, there is an individual—someone's mother, sister, friend, or partner. The narratives shared within these pages are a testament to the strength and courage of those facing breast cancer.

As an author, I acknowledge that the journey through breast cancer is ongoing. New discoveries will be made, treatments will advance, and the collective understanding of this complex condition will deepen. This work is not a final destination but rather a snapshot—a reflection of our current knowledge and a guide for the present moment.

I am grateful to the countless individuals who shared their stories, the healthcare professionals who tirelessly work to improve outcomes, and the researchers dedicated to unraveling the mysteries of breast cancer. It is through collaboration, shared experiences, and a collective commitment to progress that we can envision a future where the impact of breast cancer is diminished.

In closing, I hope this work serves as a companion, offering insights, comfort, and a sense of community to those navigating the challenges of breast cancer. It is my sincere wish that, through the power of understanding, we can collectively contribute to a world where the journey through breast cancer is marked not only by challenges but also by triumphs, resilience, and the unwavering spirit of hope.

With heartfelt sincerity,
Somtoochukwu Justin

Introduction:

Breast cancer is a formidable adversary that affects millions of women around the world. It is not just a medical condition, but a journey of resilience, strength, and, unfortunately, loss. As the author of **"Let Her Go Before Death,"** I have seen firsthand the profound effects of breast cancer on the women we love, and it is this emotional connection that has inspired me to write this book. My goal is to not only provide knowledge, but to also contribute to the ongoing dialogue surrounding breast cancer, raising awareness, fostering understanding, and offering solace.

In these pages, we will explore the various facets of breast cancer, from its causes to care, medications to considerations, risks to reduction, and the holistic approach to well-being that extends beyond the clinical setting. My hope is that this exploration will serve as both a source of information and a source of comfort for those navigating the complexities of breast cancer. Let us come together to navigate the path of understanding, compassion, and empowerment in the face of adversity.

Chapter 1: Understanding Breast Cancer

Exploring the depths of human health, breast cancer is a formidable foe that affects the lives of countless women around the world. To comprehend its impact, we must first understand the nature of breast cancer.

At its core, breast cancer is an uncontrolled growth of abnormal cells in the breast tissue. This growth usually starts in the milk-producing ducts (ductal carcinoma) or the lobules (lobular carcinoma) and can take many forms, each requiring its own diagnosis and treatment.

The cause of breast cancer is often rooted in genetic mutations. These mutations, whether inherited or acquired over time, disrupt the balance that controls cell division and growth. As a result, cells multiply uncontrollably, forming a lump in the breast, which is a sign of cancer.

The journey from healthy breast tissue to cancerous growth is a gradual process, with distinct stages. From the early stages where the tumor is still in its original place, it can spread to nearby tissues and, in more advanced cases, to other organs. Knowing these stages is essential in deciding the right course of action and creating an effective treatment plan.

Breast cancer is not one single disease, but an umbrella term for many subtypes, each with its own biological markers. These markers, such as the presence of hormone receptors (estrogen and progesterone) and the overexpression of HER2, help doctors to tailor treatments that target the cancer's specific molecular profile.

Overview of Different Types and Stages

As we explore the complexities of breast cancer, it is essential to recognize that it is not a single entity, but rather a variety of conditions, each with its own distinct characteristics. This diversity is reflected in the different types and stages of breast cancer, which can influence diagnosis, treatment, and prognosis.

When it comes to types of breast cancer, there are several to be aware of. Ductal Carcinoma In Situ (DCIS) is a non-invasive condition where abnormal cells are confined within the milk ducts, and is often seen as a precursor to invasive breast cancer. Invasive Ductal Carcinoma (IDC) is the most common form of breast cancer, and is characterized by the invasion of abnormal cells beyond the milk ducts into nearby tissues.

Lobular Carcinoma In Situ (LCIS) is an
abnormal cell growth within the lobules, which
is not considered true cancer but an indicator of
increased risk. Invasive Lobular Carcinoma
(ILC) is when cancerous cells invade the lobules
and can spread to nearby tissues.
Triple-Negative Breast Cancer lacks receptors
for estrogen, progesterone, and HER2, making it
difficult to target with hormone-based therapies.

Lastly, HER2-Positive Breast Cancer is
characterized by overexpression of the HER2
protein, often requiring targeted therapies.
Knowing the specific type is essential for
creating treatment strategies that are tailored to
the unique characteristics of the cancer.

Breast cancer staging is a system that describes
the extent of cancer spread. It is divided into
four primary stages: Stage 0 (Carcinoma In
Situ), where abnormal cells are present but have
not invaded nearby tissues; Stage I, which
involves small tumors with no lymph node

involvement; Stage II, which includes larger tumors or those with limited lymph node involvement; Stage III, which is advanced cancer with significant lymph node involvement; and Stage IV (Metastatic), where cancer has spread to distant organs.

** Statistics and Prevalence**

To truly understand the impact of breast cancer, one must look at the statistics and prevalence. These figures tell a story of the global burden that women and their communities face. Breast cancer is the most commonly diagnosed cancer among women worldwide, with millions of new cases reported each year.

Incidence rates, which reflect the number of new cases reported annually, vary from region to region. Developed countries tend to have higher rates due to increased life expectancy, lifestyle choices, and better access to healthcare.

However, the disease is on the rise in both developed and developing countries. It is important to note that men can also be diagnosed with breast cancer, though at a much lower rate. Additionally, age is a factor, as the risk increases with age. Survival rates have improved due to advances in medical research and treatment, but comprehensive care is essential for successful treatment.

Chapter 2: Causes of Breast Cancer

Unraveling the complexities of breast cancer requires us to consider a range of genetic, family history and hormonal influences. As we gain a better understanding of these factors, it becomes clear that this disease is multi-faceted.

Genetic Factors and Family History:

1. **BRCA Gene Mutations:**
   - Mutations in the BRCA1 and BRCA2 genes can significantly increase the risk of breast cancer. Those who inherit these mutations from their parents are more likely to develop the disease.

2. **Family History:**
   - A family history of breast cancer may be indicative of shared genetic predispositions or environmental factors. Women with a first-degree relative (mother, sister, or daughter)

who have been diagnosed with breast cancer are at an increased risk.

3. **Inherited Genetic Syndromes:**
   - Certain inherited syndromes, such as Li-Fraumeni syndrome and Cowden syndrome, are associated with a heightened risk of breast cancer.

4. **Personal Genetic Makeup:**
   - In addition to well-known genetic mutations, variations in many other genes can contribute to individual susceptibility. Research is ongoing to better understand these genetic intricacies.

Gaining insight into the genetic basis of breast cancer can help with risk assessment, as well as preventive measures and personalized treatment approaches.

Hormonal Influences:

1. **Estrogen and Progesterone Receptors:**

- Breast cancer growth is often influenced by hormonal receptors on the surface of cancer cells. Tumors that express estrogen receptors (ER-positive) or progesterone receptors (PR-positive) can respond to hormonal therapies.

2. **Hormone Replacement Therapy (HRT):**
   - Long-term use of hormone replacement therapy, particularly estrogen-progestin combinations during menopause, has been linked to an increased risk of breast cancer.

3. **Early Menstruation and Late Menopause:**
   - Women who experience menstruation at an early age or undergo menopause later in life are exposed to a longer period of hormonal fluctuations, which may increase their risk.

4. **Pregnancy and Breastfeeding:**
   - Early childbirth and prolonged breastfeeding can have a protective effect, reducing exposure to hormonal fluctuations associated with breast cancer.

Lifestyle Factors: Diet and Physical Activity**

In the complex tapestry of breast cancer causation, lifestyle factors are key threads. Our daily choices can have a direct impact on our risk of developing this pervasive disease. Diet and physical activity are two areas where proactive measures can be taken to reduce the risk of breast cancer.

When it comes to diet, high-fat diets, such as those found in red meat and full-fat dairy products, have been linked to an increased risk. On the other hand, diets rich in lean proteins, fruits, vegetables, and whole grains may offer protective benefits. Additionally, alcohol consumption has been linked to an increased risk of breast cancer, so moderation or abstention is often recommended.

Fruits and vegetables, which are full of antioxidants and vitamins, can also help reduce the risk. Finally, maintaining a healthy weight is important, as obesity is a known risk factor, particularly in postmenopausal women.

Physical activity is also important for reducing the risk of breast cancer. Regular exercise, such as brisk walking, jogging, or other aerobic exercises, can help. The benefits of physical activity extend into the postmenopausal years, and consistency is key - long-term engagement in physical activity appears to have a more substantial impact.

Environmental Factors and Toxic Exposures**

As we continue to investigate the complex causes of breast cancer, it is becoming increasingly clear that our environment plays a major role in determining our health outcomes. In this section, we will explore the impact of environmental factors and toxic exposures, and how they can contribute to the multifaceted nature of breast cancer.

Endocrine Disruptors: Exposure to certain endocrine-disrupting chemicals, found in plastics, pesticides, and industrial pollutants, has been linked to an increased risk of breast cancer. These substances can interfere with hormonal balance and may be a factor in the development of hormone-sensitive tumors.

Radiation Exposure: Prolonged exposure to ionizing radiation, whether from medical procedures or environmental sources, is a known risk factor for breast cancer. It is essential that we take steps to reduce unnecessary radiation exposure and ensure safety in medical settings.

Air Pollution: Recent research has suggested a potential connection between long-term exposure to air pollution and an elevated risk of breast cancer. It is important that we address and reduce sources of air pollution, not only for breast health, but for overall well-being.

Occupational Exposures: Certain occupations may involve exposure to carcinogens or endocrine-disrupting chemicals, which could increase the risk of breast cancer. It is important to be aware of workplace safety and use protective measures when necessary.

Chemical Contaminants: Chemical contaminants in water, soil, and consumer products have raised questions about their potential contribution to breast cancer risk. It is essential that we monitor and regulate exposure to these contaminants for the sake of public health.

Personal Care Products: Some ingredients in personal care products, such as certain parabens and phthalates, have been linked to breast cancer. It may be wise to choose products with minimal chemical additives and opt for alternatives when possible.

Chapter 3: Breast Cancer Care and Diagnosis

In the fight against breast cancer, regular screenings are essential for early detection and successful treatment. This chapter highlights the importance of screenings, emphasizing their role in timely diagnosis and effective intervention.

Importance of Regular Screenings:

1. **Early Detection Saves Lives:**
   - Regular screenings, such as mammograms and clinical breast exams, are proactive measures to detect abnormalities in their earliest stages. Early detection increases the chances of successful treatment and long-term survival.

2. **Identification of Precancerous Lesions:**
   - Screenings not only detect invasive breast cancers but also identify precancerous lesions, allowing for preventive measures and interventions before cancer fully develops.

3. **Tailoring Treatment Approaches:**
   - Timely detection provides healthcare professionals with valuable information to customize treatment plans according to the specific characteristics of the cancer. This personalized approach enhances the effectiveness of interventions.

4. **Reducing Treatment Intensity:**
   - Early-stage breast cancers often require less aggressive treatments, minimizing the physical and emotional impact on individuals. This underscores the importance of early detection in optimizing treatment outcomes.

Screening Modalities:

1. **Mammography:**
   - Mammograms, X-ray images of the breast, are a standard screening tool for breast cancer. Regular mammography is recommended, especially for women aged 40 and older, to

detect abnormalities that may not be palpable during a clinical exam.

2. **Clinical Breast Exams:**
   - Regular clinical breast exams conducted by healthcare professionals complement mammography. These hands-on examinations help identify changes in breast tissue texture and structure.

3. **Breast Self-Exams:**
   - While breast self-exams are not a substitute for professional screenings, they empower individuals to become familiar with their bodies. Any changes or abnormalities detected during self-exams should prompt consultation with a healthcare provider.

The Power of Knowledge:

1. **Educating and Empowering Individuals:**
   - Raising awareness about the importance of screenings empowers individuals to take charge of their breast health. Knowledgeable and

proactive engagement with healthcare providers fosters a culture of preventive care.

2. **Addressing Disparities:**
   - Advocacy for equitable access to screenings is paramount in addressing disparities in breast cancer outcomes. Initiatives that increase awareness and facilitate screenings in underserved communities contribute to closing gaps in healthcare access.

Overview of Diagnostic Procedures

As we explore the world of breast cancer care, diagnostic procedures are the key to uncovering the complexities of the disease. This section provides an overview of the main diagnostic procedures, helping to confirm diagnoses and create personalized treatment plans.

Mammography:

1. **Purpose and Procedure:**
   - Mammography is an X-ray of the breast tissue and is a fundamental part of breast cancer diagnosis. It can detect abnormalities such as lumps or microcalcifications that may suggest the presence of cancer.

2. **Screening vs. Diagnostic Mammograms:**
   - Screening mammograms are routine tests for people without symptoms, while diagnostic mammograms are used when abnormalities are found or when there are breast-related

Let her go before death

symptoms. Both are essential for the diagnostic process.

Breast Ultrasound:

1. **Purpose and Procedure:**
   - Ultrasound imaging uses sound waves to create a detailed image of the breast tissue. It is often used as an additional tool to investigate abnormalities seen in mammograms or physical exams.

2. **Guidance for Biopsies:**
   - Breast ultrasound can help guide the placement of a needle during biopsy procedures, ensuring accurate sampling of suspicious tissue.

Breast Biopsy:

1. **Types of Biopsies:**
   - Biopsies involve taking a small tissue sample for examination under a microscope. Common biopsy types include core needle biopsy, fine-needle aspiration, and surgical biopsy.

2. **Definitive Diagnosis:**
   - A biopsy provides a definitive diagnosis by analyzing the tissue for the presence of cancer cells. This information is essential for determining the type, grade, and molecular characteristics of the cancer.

MRI (Magnetic Resonance Imaging):

1. **Purpose and Application:**
   - Breast MRI uses magnetic fields and radio waves to create detailed images of the breast tissue. It is often used in specific situations, such as assessing the extent of cancer or evaluating high-risk individuals.

2. **Enhancing Treatment Planning:**
   - MRI findings provide valuable information for treatment planning, helping healthcare professionals tailor interventions to the unique characteristics of the cancer.

Genetic Testing:

Identification of Genetic Mutations:
  - Genetic testing looks for mutations in certain genes, such as BRCA1 and BRCA2. Positive results can influence treatment decisions and provide preventive measures for people at a higher risk.

** The Emotional Impact of Receiving a Diagnosis**

The moment a person is diagnosed with breast cancer is a life-changing experience. This chapter explores the emotional complexities that come with this pivotal moment, and the immediate impact it has on individuals and their loved ones.

Shock and Disbelief:
When someone is diagnosed with breast cancer, they may be overcome with shock and disbelief. The sudden realization of mortality and the reality of a life-altering condition can be overwhelming. People may struggle to comprehend the news, and the gravity of the diagnosis.

Fear and Anxiety:
Fear of the unknown and anxiety about the future can become constant companions. Questions about treatment options, potential

outcomes, and the effect on daily life can flood the mind. The uncertainty of the journey ahead can cause profound anxiety, for both the person diagnosed and their support network.

Grief and Loss:
A breast cancer diagnosis brings with it a sense of grief and loss—for the life one had envisioned, for a sense of control over one's health, and for the perceived invincibility that may have existed before the diagnosis. Coping with these losses is an important part of the emotional journey.

Anger and Frustration:
Feelings of anger and frustration are common reactions to a breast cancer diagnosis. Anger may be directed at the perceived injustice of the situation or frustration with the limitations the diagnosis imposes. Navigating these emotions is a dynamic process that evolves over time.

Impact on Relationships:

The emotional impact extends to relationships with family and friends. Loved ones often share in the emotional turbulence, feeling helpless, scared, and sad. Open communication and mutual support are essential in managing the complexities of these relationships.

Coping Mechanisms:
Individuals diagnosed with breast cancer often develop coping mechanisms to manage the emotional storm. This may include seeking solace in support groups, relying on spiritual or religious beliefs, or finding comfort in creative outlets. Understanding and embracing these coping mechanisms can help build emotional resilience.

Hope and Resilience:
Amidst the emotional turmoil, hope and resilience can be found. Many individuals find strength in connecting with others who have faced similar challenges, and the journey itself often becomes a testament to the strength of the human spirit.

Chapter 4: Treatment Options

Navigating the path of breast cancer treatment requires a personalized approach, tailored to the individual's diagnosis. This chapter provides an overview of the key treatment modalities—surgery, chemotherapy, radiation therapy, and hormonal therapy—that form the foundation of breast cancer care.

Surgery:

1. **Lumpectomy:**
   - This surgical procedure involves removing the tumor along with a margin of healthy tissue surrounding it. Lumpectomy is often an option for early-stage breast cancer.

2. **Mastectomy:**
   - This is the removal of the entire breast and may be recommended for larger tumors, certain

types of breast cancer, or when a person chooses
a more aggressive approach.

3. **Sentinel Lymph Node Biopsy:**
   - During surgery, the sentinel lymph node, the
first node to which cancer cells are likely to
spread, may be removed and examined to
determine if cancer has spread beyond the
primary site.

Chemotherapy:

1. **Purpose and Administration:**
   - Chemotherapy uses powerful drugs to
destroy or inhibit the growth of cancer cells. It
can be administered orally or intravenously and
is often recommended to target cancer cells
throughout the body.

2. **Neoadjuvant and Adjuvant Therapy:**
   - Neoadjuvant chemotherapy is given before
surgery to shrink tumors, while adjuvant
chemotherapy is administered after surgery to

eliminate any remaining cancer cells and reduce the risk of recurrence.

Radiation Therapy:

1. **Purpose and Techniques:**
   - Radiation therapy uses high-energy rays to target and destroy cancer cells. It is commonly employed after surgery to eliminate any remaining cancer cells and reduce the risk of local recurrence.

2. **External Beam vs. Internal Radiation:**
   - External beam radiation delivers radiation from outside the body, while internal radiation (brachytherapy) involves placing a radiation source inside or very close to the tumor.

Hormonal Therapy:

1. **Purpose and Target Population:**
   - Hormonal therapy is primarily used for hormone receptor-positive breast cancers. It

works by blocking hormones that fuel certain types of breast cancer.

2. **Tamoxifen and Aromatase Inhibitors:**
   - Tamoxifen is a commonly prescribed hormonal therapy for both premenopausal and postmenopausal women. Aromatase inhibitors, typically used in postmenopausal women, reduce estrogen production.

Immunotherapy and Targeted Therapies:

1. **Immunotherapy:**
   - Immunotherapy is an emerging field in breast cancer treatment, which uses the body's immune system to recognize and eliminate cancer cells.

2. **Targeted Therapies:**
   - Targeted therapies focus on specific molecular characteristics of cancer cells, such as HER2-positive breast cancers. These drugs aim to disrupt specific pathways involved in cancer growth.

Personalized Treatment Plans

The field of breast cancer treatment has changed drastically, now recognizing the individual needs of each patient. Personalized treatment plans, tailored to the specific characteristics of the cancer and the person's overall health, have become the norm in modern oncology. This chapter will discuss the components and importance of personalized treatment in the fight against breast cancer.

Understanding Tumor Characteristics:

1. Tumor Type and Subtype:
   - Identifying the type and subtype of breast cancer, such as hormone receptor status (estrogen and progesterone receptors) and HER2 expression, is essential for making treatment decisions.

2. Genetic Profiling:
   - Advances in genetic testing allow for a deeper understanding of the genetic makeup of

the tumor. This information helps predict how the cancer may behave and assists in creating tailored treatment strategies.

Tailoring Treatment Modalities:

1. Surgery:
  - Personalized treatment plans determine the extent of surgical intervention, choosing between lumpectomy and mastectomy based on the size and characteristics of the tumor.

2. Chemotherapy:
  - The decision to use chemotherapy, the specific drugs employed, and the timing of administration are all individualized based on factors such as tumor size, lymph node involvement, and genetic characteristics.

3. Radiation Therapy:
  - Personalized plans assess the necessity and duration of radiation therapy, considering factors like the extent of surgery, lymph node status, and overall health.

4. Hormonal Therapy:
   - Hormonal therapy choices are influenced by hormone receptor status, with medications like tamoxifen or aromatase inhibitors prescribed based on menopausal status and individual risk factors.

5. Targeted Therapies:
   - Personalized treatment may incorporate targeted therapies, especially for HER2-positive breast cancers. These therapies specifically address the molecular characteristics of the cancer cells.

Considering Overall Health and Preferences:

1. Patient Preferences:
   - Personalized treatment plans take into account the individual's values, preferences, and lifestyle. Shared decision-making between patients and healthcare providers ensures a treatment approach that is in line with the patient's goals.

2. Overall Health and Comorbidities:
   - The person's overall health, including pre-existing conditions and comorbidities, is a crucial factor in tailoring treatment plans. Adjustments may be made to ensure the overall well-being of the individual.

Monitoring and Adjusting:

1. Response Monitoring:
   - Ongoing assessment of treatment response through imaging, blood tests, and clinical exams informs adjustments to the treatment plan as needed.

2. Adapting to Changes:
   - Personalized treatment plans are dynamic and adaptable. Changes may be made based on treatment response, emerging research, or the development of new therapeutic options.

The introduction of personalized treatment plans marks a major shift in breast cancer care, recognizing the uniqueness of each person's journey.

Side Effects and Coping Mechanisms

Beginning the journey of breast cancer treatment is a courageous and life-changing experience. However, it can come with a range of physical and emotional side effects. This chapter will discuss the common side effects associated with various treatments, as well as provide effective coping mechanisms to help individuals manage the challenges of breast cancer.

Common Treatment Side Effects:

1. **Fatigue:**
   - Fatigue is a common symptom that can be caused by the cumulative effects of surgery, chemotherapy, radiation, and hormonal therapy.

2. **Nausea and Vomiting:**
   - Nausea and vomiting are often associated with chemotherapy, but anti-nausea medications can help manage these symptoms.

3. **Hair Loss:**
   - Some chemotherapy drugs may lead to temporary hair loss. Wigs, scarves, or embracing one's natural appearance can be empowering.

4. **Changes in Skin and Nails:**
   - Radiation therapy and certain medications can cause skin and nail changes. Gentle skincare practices and protective measures can help alleviate discomfort.

5. **Cognitive Changes (Chemo Brain):**
   - Some individuals may experience cognitive changes, often referred to as "chemo brain." Cognitive exercises, organization strategies, and adequate rest can help mitigate these effects.

6. **Menopausal Symptoms:**
   - Hormonal therapy, especially in postmenopausal women, can induce symptoms such as hot flashes and mood swings. Lifestyle adjustments and medications can help manage these symptoms.

Emotional and Psychological Effects:

1. **Anxiety and Depression:**
   - The weight of a breast cancer diagnosis and treatment can contribute to anxiety and depression. Counseling, support groups, and mindfulness practices can offer emotional support.

2. **Body Image Concerns:**
   - Changes in physical appearance, such as hair loss and surgical alterations, can affect body image. Support from loved ones and counseling services can help with these concerns.

3. **Fear of Recurrence:**
   - The fear of cancer recurrence is a common emotional challenge. Open communication with healthcare providers, support groups, and mental health professionals can help alleviate this fear.

Coping Mechanisms:

1. **Support Systems:**
   - Building a strong support system, including family, friends, and support groups, can provide emotional and practical assistance throughout the journey.

2. **Mind-Body Practices:**
   - Incorporating mind-body practices such as meditation, yoga, and deep-breathing exercises can promote relaxation and mental well-being.

3. **Creative Outlets:**
   - Engaging in creative activities, like art, writing, or music, can provide an expressive outlet and a sense of accomplishment.

4. **Nutrition and Exercise:**
   - Eating a balanced diet and exercising regularly can contribute to physical and emotional well-being. Consulting with healthcare providers ensures alignment with individual health needs.

5. **Communication with Healthcare Providers:**
   - Open and honest communication with healthcare providers about side effects allows for timely interventions and adjustments to the treatment plan.

Chapter 5: Medications in Breast Cancer Treatment

The range of drugs used to treat breast cancer is vast, reflecting the complexity of the disease. This chapter provides an overview of the key medications used in various treatments, such as chemotherapy, hormonal therapy, targeted therapies, and supportive medications. It is important to understand the purpose and potential side effects of each medication in order to make informed decisions and manage breast cancer effectively.

Chemotherapy medications include doxorubicin (Adriamycin), a powerful anthracycline drug used in combination with other drugs; cyclophosphamide (Cytoxan), which interferes with cancer cell growth; and paclitaxel (Taxol) and docetaxel (Taxotere), taxane drugs that disrupt cell division.

Hormonal therapy medications include tamoxifen, a selective estrogen receptor modulator (SERM) used in pre- and postmenopausal women with hormone receptor-positive breast cancer; aromatase inhibitors (Anastrozole, Letrozole, Exemestane), which reduce estrogen levels; and fulvestrant (Faslodex), an estrogen receptor antagonist used in advanced hormone receptor-positive breast cancer.

Targeted therapy medications include trastuzumab (Herceptin), a monoclonal antibody that targets the HER2 protein; and lapatinib (Tykerb), an oral medication that targets both HER2 and EGFR receptors. Immunotherapy medications include pembrolizumab (Keytruda), which may be used in certain cases of triple-negative breast cancer. Bone-modifying agents include zoledronic acid (Zometa) and denosumab (Xgeva), which are used to strengthen bones and reduce the risk of fractures in individuals with breast cancer that has spread to the bones.

Supportive medications include antiemetics, such as ondansetron (Zofran) and aprepitant (Emend), which help manage chemotherapy-induced nausea and vomiting; and granulocyte-colony stimulating factor (G-CSF) drugs, such as filgrastim (Neupogen) and pegfilgrastim (Neulasta), which stimulate the production of white blood cells and reduce the risk of infection during chemotherapy.

** The Crucial Importance of Adherence to Prescribed Medications**

Adhering to prescribed medications is essential for successful breast cancer treatment. This chapter will explore the critical importance of adherence, and how it can affect treatment efficacy, prevent complications, and improve overall well-being throughout the breast cancer journey.

Optimizing treatment efficacy is one of the main benefits of adhering to medications. Consistent and timely administration of therapeutic agents helps to ensure that they have their intended effect on cancer cells, and can help to stop or shrink the tumor.

Adherence is also important for preventing disease progression. Interruptions or irregularities in medication regimens can give cancer cells the opportunity to become resistant or spread, which can compromise the effectiveness of the treatment plan.

Post-treatment medications, such as hormonal therapies, can help to reduce the risk of cancer recurrence. Taking these medications as prescribed is essential for achieving this goal.

Adherence also allows healthcare providers to monitor and manage potential side effects. Timely intervention can help to reduce discomfort and prevent complications, so that individuals can continue their treatment with minimal disruption.

Adherence can also improve quality of life during and after treatment. By minimizing disease-related symptoms and preventing complications, individuals can better maintain their daily activities, work, and overall well-being.

The emotional toll of a breast cancer diagnosis and treatment journey can be immense.

Adherence can provide a sense of control and empowerment, which can positively influence mental and emotional well-being. Knowing that one is actively participating in their treatment plan can help to foster a resilient mindset.

Adherence also builds trust between individuals and their healthcare providers. A collaborative approach, where individuals understand the importance of adherence and healthcare providers actively support and address concerns, can help to foster a positive therapeutic relationship.

Regular and consistent adherence is also key for preventing the development of medication resistance. This is especially important in breast cancer, where resistance can arise and limit the effectiveness of certain treatments over time.

Adhering to prescribed medications can also help to improve long-term outcomes. Whether it's hormonal therapy, targeted therapies, or supportive medications, consistent use can help to achieve and sustain remission.

Finally, adherence empowers individuals to actively participate in their health journey. Understanding the importance of each medication and its role in the treatment plan can help to enhance a sense of agency, and foster a proactive approach to health and recovery.

Chapter 6: Risks and Risk Reduction in Breast Cancer

It is important to understand the various factors that can contribute to the risk of developing breast cancer in order to take proactive steps to manage one's health. This chapter will explore the various risk factors associated with breast cancer and discuss strategies for reducing the risk and taking preventive measures.

Genetic Factors and Family History: A family history of breast cancer, particularly if it involves a first-degree relative (mother, sister, or daughter), and the presence of specific genetic mutations (BRCA1, BRCA2) can increase the risk of breast cancer.

Hormonal Influences: Prolonged exposure to estrogen, such as early onset of menstruation, late onset of menopause, or hormone replacement therapy, can increase the risk of hormone receptor-positive breast cancers.

Age: The risk of breast cancer increases with age, with the majority of cases diagnosed in women over the age of 50.

Gender: While breast cancer is much more common in women, men can also develop the disease, albeit at a lower incidence.

Personal History of Breast Cancer or Certain Non-Cancerous Breast Diseases: People who have previously had breast cancer or certain non-cancerous breast diseases may have an elevated risk of developing a new cancer.

Lifestyle Factors: Unhealthy lifestyle choices, such as excessive alcohol consumption, smoking, a diet high in processed foods, and lack of physical activity, can increase the risk of breast cancer.

Reproductive History: Delayed childbirth, having fewer children, or not breastfeeding may contribute to an increased risk of breast cancer.

Radiation Exposure: Previous exposure to radiation, especially during certain medical procedures like chest X-rays or radiation therapy, can elevate the risk of developing breast cancer.

Environmental Factors: While the impact of environmental factors is still under investigation, exposure to certain substances like endocrine-disrupting chemicals and pollutants may contribute to an increased risk.

In order to reduce the risk of breast cancer, it is important to take preventive measures tailored to each person's health profile. Regular mammograms and clinical breast exams can facilitate early detection, enabling timely intervention and reducing the impact of the disease.

Hormonal therapies such as tamoxifen or aromatase inhibitors may be recommended to reduce the risk of hormone receptor-positive breast cancers. Adopting a healthy lifestyle, including a balanced diet, regular exercise, limited alcohol consumption, and avoidance of smoking, can help reduce the risk of breast cancer. Individuals with a family history of breast cancer may benefit from genetic counseling and testing to identify specific genetic mutations and inform risk reduction strategies.

Certain medications, such as tamoxifen or raloxifene, may be considered for women at increased risk to reduce the likelihood of developing breast cancer. In some high-risk cases, prophylactic surgery (mastectomy) may be considered to reduce the risk of breast cancer.

Empowering Lifestyle Changes for Breast Cancer Risk Reduction

Taking charge of one's health through lifestyle changes is a proactive and empowering way to reduce the risk of breast cancer. This chapter looks at practical lifestyle modifications that individuals can make to promote overall well-being and lower the risk of developing breast cancer.

1. Plant-Based Diet:
  - **Fruits and Veggies:** Eating plenty of fruits and vegetables provides essential vitamins, minerals, and antioxidants. These nutrients help support overall health and may help reduce cancer risk.
  - **Whole Grains and Lean Proteins:** Choose whole grains and lean protein sources to maintain a balanced and nutritious diet.

2. Regular Exercise:
  - **Cardio:** Engage in regular cardiovascular exercise such as walking,

jogging, or cycling. Aim for at least 150 minutes of moderate-intensity exercise per week.

- **Strength Training:** Include strength training exercises at least two days a week to enhance muscle strength and overall fitness.

3. Healthy Weight:

- **Body Mass Index (BMI):** Aim for a healthy body weight within the recommended BMI range. Maintaining a healthy weight is associated with a lower risk of breast cancer.

- **Balanced Diet and Exercise:** Combine a balanced diet with regular physical activity to achieve and sustain a healthy weight.

4. Limiting Alcohol:

- **Moderation:** Limit alcohol intake to moderate levels—up to one drink per day for women. Excessive alcohol consumption is linked to an increased risk of breast cancer.

5. Quitting Smoking:

- **Cessation:** Quitting smoking is a crucial step in reducing the risk of various health issues, including breast cancer.

6. Breastfeeding:
   - **Benefits:** If possible, consider breastfeeding. It not only provides numerous health benefits for the child but also reduces the mother's risk of breast cancer.

7. Mindful Hormone Replacement Therapy (HRT):
   - **Informed Decision-Making:** If considering hormone replacement therapy for menopausal symptoms, engage in open discussions with healthcare providers about potential risks and benefits. Make informed decisions based on individual health considerations.

8. Stress Management:
   - **Mindfulness Practices:** Incorporate stress-reducing techniques into daily life, such as meditation, yoga, or deep-breathing exercises.

Managing stress is essential for overall well-being.

9. Regular Health Check-ups and Screenings:
  - **Early Detection:** Schedule regular health check-ups and breast cancer screenings, including mammograms. Early detection allows for timely intervention and better outcomes.

10. Genetic Counseling and Testing:
  - **Understanding Genetic Risk:** Individuals with a family history of breast cancer can benefit from genetic counseling and testing. Knowing one's genetic risk can guide personalized risk reduction strategies.

The Crucial Importance of Regular Check-ups and Screenings

Regular health check-ups and screenings are essential for breast cancer prevention and early detection. This chapter highlights the importance of routine medical examinations and screenings, emphasizing their role in preserving overall health and increasing the likelihood of successful outcomes in breast cancer care.

Early detection is key to saving lives: timely intervention through regular mammograms can detect breast cancer in its earliest stages, allowing for more effective and less aggressive treatment options. Screenings can also identify precancerous changes or lesions, providing an opportunity to intervene before they progress to invasive cancer.

For individuals with a family history of breast cancer or known genetic mutations, regular check-ups and screenings allow for close monitoring and early detection. This increases the likelihood of successful treatment outcomes, as early intervention often allows for less invasive treatments and preserves more of the breast. Additionally, early detection is associated with higher survival rates, as it catches potential issues at their most treatable stages.

Regular check-ups also provide opportunities for healthcare providers to tailor personalized treatment plans based on the individual's health status, risk factors, and response to previous treatments. Furthermore, they allow for the timely management of potential complications related to breast cancer or its treatments, minimizing the impact on overall health.

For women, regular check-ups encompass a comprehensive well-woman care approach, addressing reproductive health, cardiovascular health, and other aspects of overall wellness. They also offer opportunities for health education, empowering individuals to make informed choices about lifestyle, diet, and preventive measures.

Overall, regular check-ups foster a proactive health mindset, encouraging individuals to actively engage in their health care and advocate for their well-being.

Chapter 7: Age and Breast Cancer: Understanding the Risk Dynamics

Age is a major factor in the complicated landscape of breast cancer risk. This chapter examines the connection between age and breast cancer, looking at the age ranges associated with higher risk and the dynamic considerations for screening and preventive measures.

Postmenopausal women are particularly at risk for breast cancer, with the majority of cases being diagnosed in women over the age of 50. Breast cancer incidence gradually increases with age, with the highest rates seen in women over 70. However, younger women are not immune to the risk of breast cancer, so vigilance and awareness are essential for all women.

Younger women with a family history of breast cancer or certain genetic mutations may be at an increased risk. Genetic counseling and testing may be recommended in such cases. Additionally, reproductive factors such as early onset of menstruation, late onset of menopause, and not having children can influence breast cancer risk in younger women.

The relationship between age and hormone receptor status (estrogen receptor-positive, progesterone receptor-positive) can also affect treatment decisions and outcomes. Mammography is a key tool for breast cancer detection, and screening guidelines may vary based on age. Breast tissue changes with age, which can affect the accuracy of mammograms, so radiologists take breast density and composition into account when interpreting results.

Individualized screening approaches should be taken into account, considering factors such as family history, genetic predisposition, and personal health history. Postmenopausal women should discuss the risks and benefits of hormone replacement therapy (HRT) with their healthcare providers, as HRT is associated with increased breast cancer risk. Age also influences survivorship considerations, as older survivors may face unique challenges related to comorbidities, treatment tolerability, and quality of life.

Finally, regardless of age, healthy lifestyle choices, such as a balanced diet and regular physical activity, can contribute to overall well-being and may impact breast cancer risk.

Age-Appropriate Screenings and Empowering Awareness

Tailoring breast cancer screenings to specific age groups is essential for effective detection and prevention. This chapter focuses on age-appropriate screenings and emphasizes the importance of raising awareness across different stages of life.

Women in their 20s and 30s should have a clinical breast exam as part of a routine health examination at least every three years. It is also important to develop breast self-awareness and understand normal breast changes. Any changes or concerns should be reported to healthcare providers promptly.

Beginning in their 40s, women are encouraged to have annual mammograms. Mammography is a key tool for detecting breast cancer at an early, more treatable stage. Regular clinical breast exams by healthcare professionals should also continue, complementing mammography.

Women in their 50s should continue with annual mammograms, providing ongoing surveillance for potential breast abnormalities. Regular health check-ups become increasingly important, addressing overall well-being and potential age-related health concerns.

Mammograms remain a crucial part of breast cancer screening for women over 60. Regular screenings contribute to maintaining breast health in the later stages of life. Tailoring screening recommendations based on an individual's health status, life expectancy, and preferences becomes more relevant.

Breast cancer survivors of all ages should remain vigilant about post-treatment monitoring, including regular follow-up appointments and screenings. Emphasizing healthy lifestyle choices, including regular exercise and a balanced diet, is particularly important for long-term survivorship.

Women with a family history of breast cancer or specific genetic mutations may benefit from genetic counseling and testing at any age.

Encouraging breast health awareness through educational initiatives, community programs, and outreach efforts is essential. This includes understanding the importance of screenings and knowing how to perform breast self-exams. Providing women with comprehensive information about breast cancer risk, screenings, and preventive measures empowers them to make informed decisions about their health.

Women transitioning through menopause should discuss the risks and benefits of hormone replacement therapy (HRT) with their healthcare providers, considering its potential impact on breast cancer risk.

Ongoing education and advocacy efforts within communities help raise awareness about the importance of age-appropriate screenings, early detection, and overall breast health. Embracing digital tools and resources, including mobile applications and online platforms, can enhance breast health awareness and facilitate access to relevant information.

By aligning screenings with age-appropriate guidelines and raising awareness at different life stages, individuals can actively participate in their breast health. Regular discussions with healthcare providers and engagement in educational initiatives contribute to a proactive approach to breast cancer prevention.

Chapter 8: Navigating Toxic Exposure: Unraveling the Environmental Links to Breast Cancer

Comprehending the effect of toxic exposure on the risk of breast cancer is a vital part of comprehensive breast health awareness. This chapter examines the intricate relationship between environmental factors and the potential connections to the development of breast cancer.

Environmental Factors and Breast Cancer Risk:
  - **Complex Interplay:** The risk of breast cancer is affected by a complex combination of genetic, hormonal, and environmental factors. Environmental exposures are part of this multifaceted landscape.

Endocrine-Disrupting Chemicals (EDCs):
  - **Altering Hormone Function:** EDCs, found in various household products, plastics,

and pesticides, have the potential to interfere with hormonal balance. Prolonged exposure to these chemicals may lead to an increased risk of breast cancer.

Pesticides and Herbicides:
   - **Agricultural Impact:** Women living in agricultural areas or those working in farming may be exposed to higher levels of pesticides and herbicides, which have been associated with an elevated risk of breast cancer.

Occupational Exposures:
   - **Workplace Risks:** Certain occupational environments involve exposure to substances linked to breast cancer, such as certain solvents, heavy metals, and industrial chemicals.

Air Pollution and Urban Living:
   - **Residential Impact:** Urban living and exposure to air pollution have been explored as potential contributors to breast cancer risk. Knowing these links is essential, especially for women living in densely populated areas.

Plastics and Bisphenol A (BPA):
 - **Everyday Exposure:** Plastics containing BPA, commonly found in food and beverage containers, may pose risks. BPA is an endocrine-disrupting chemical, and its potential effect on breast cancer risk is an area of ongoing research.

Personal Care Products:
 - **Chemical Ingredients:** Some personal care products contain chemicals that may act as endocrine disruptors. Regular and prolonged use of these products may lead to cumulative exposure.

Radiation Exposure:
 - **Medical Procedures:** Certain medical procedures involving ionizing radiation, such as chest X-rays or CT scans, may contribute to breast cancer risk. While the benefits of these procedures often outweigh the risks, minimizing unnecessary exposure is essential.

Lifestyle Choices and Environmental Impact:
   - **Consumer Decisions:** Lifestyle choices, including diet and consumer habits, can influence exposure to potential carcinogens. Adopting eco-friendly practices may contribute to both environmental and personal well-being.

Geographic Variances in Exposure:
   - **Regional Influences:** An individual's geographic location can affect exposure levels. Knowing regional variances in environmental factors is crucial for assessing breast cancer risk.

Advocacy for Environmental Health:
   - **Community Awareness:** Supporting policies that prioritize environmental health and participating in community initiatives can contribute to broader efforts in reducing toxic exposures and promoting breast health.

Breast Cancer Prevention through Environmental Awareness:
   - **Informed Decision-Making:** Making informed decisions about lifestyle choices,

product usage, and environmental exposures allows individuals to actively participate in breast cancer prevention.

Nurturing Health: Minimizing Toxin Exposure in Daily Life

Empowering individuals with the tools to reduce their daily toxin exposure is essential for promoting overall health and wellbeing. This chapter looks at proactive steps and lifestyle choices that can help minimize exposure to environmental toxins.

1. Conscious Consumer Choices:
- **Read Labels:** Carefully read labels on personal care products, household cleaners, and cosmetics. Choose items with fewer chemicals and toxins, and pick products from companies that are transparent.

2. Choose Natural and Organic Products:
- **Go Natural:** Whenever possible, opt for natural and organic products. This includes food, cleaning supplies, and personal care items. Look for certifications that indicate organic or eco-friendly standards.

3. Limit Plastic Usage:
- **Switch to Glass or Stainless Steel:** Use glass or stainless steel containers for food and beverages. Minimize the use of plastic containers, especially those with recycling codes that could indicate harmful substances.

4. Filter Drinking Water:
- **Invest in a Water Filter:** Use a water filter to reduce exposure to contaminants in tap water. This is especially important in areas where water quality may be a concern.

5. Mindful Food Choices:
- **Choose Organic Produce:** Opt for organic fruits and vegetables to reduce exposure to pesticides. Clean conventionally grown produce thoroughly to remove residues.
- **Select Hormone-Free Meats:** Choose meats that are raised without the use of hormones or antibiotics to minimize potential chemical exposure.

6. Ventilation in Living Spaces:
- **Ensure Adequate Ventilation:** Make sure there is proper ventilation in living spaces to reduce indoor air pollution. Open windows regularly, use air purifiers, and avoid the use of certain indoor pollutants.

7. Be Mindful of Personal Care Products:
- **Simplify Beauty Routines:** Limit the use of cosmetics and personal care products with a long list of ingredients. Simplify beauty routines to reduce exposure to unnecessary chemicals.

8. Mind Your Cleaning Products:
- **Make Homemade Cleaning Solutions:** Consider using homemade cleaning solutions with natural ingredients like vinegar, baking soda, and lemon. Alternatively, choose eco-friendly cleaning products.

9. Practice Safe Food Storage:
- **Avoid Plastic Containers for Heating:** Avoid using plastic containers for heating food

in microwaves, as heat can cause chemicals to
leach into the food.

10. Choose Safer Cookware:
- **Go for Non-Toxic Cookware:** Opt for
non-toxic cookware, such as stainless steel, cast
iron, or ceramic. Be mindful of potential risks
associated with non-stick coatings.

11. Mindful Use of Electronics:
- **Reduce Exposure to EMFs:** Minimize
exposure to electromagnetic fields (EMFs) from
electronic devices. Keep mobile phones away
from the body, use speakerphone or earphones,
and turn off devices when not in use.

12. Natural Pest Control:
- **Avoid Harsh Pesticides:** Choose natural
and non-toxic methods for pest control in and
around the home. This includes using traps,
barriers, and natural repellents.

13. Regular Detoxification Practices:

- **Support the Body's Natural Detoxification:** Incorporate practices that support the body's natural detoxification processes. This includes staying hydrated, consuming detoxifying foods, and engaging in activities like saunas or sweating exercises.

14. Stay Informed and Advocate:
- **Raise Community Awareness:** Stay informed about environmental issues in your community. Advocate for policies that prioritize environmental health and participate in community initiatives focused on reducing toxins.

Chapter 9: Unveiling the Connection: Chronic Inflammation and Cancer Risk

The relationship between chronic inflammation and cancer is a complex and dynamic interplay that requires further exploration. This chapter will delve into the intricate connections between long-term inflammation and the increased risk of cancer, with a particular focus on breast cancer.

Normal immune response involves inflammation, which is a natural and essential part of the immune system's response to injury or infection. Chronic inflammation, however, is when the immune system is persistently activated, leading to a prolonged release of inflammatory signals and mediators. This can cause cellular changes that create an environment conducive to the development and progression of cancer, as well as DNA damage and mutations, increasing the likelihood of uncontrolled cell growth.

In terms of breast cancer, inflammation in breast tissue may play a role in its development, particularly in cases of long-term inflammation. Persistent infections, such as certain viral or bacterial infections, as well as autoimmune diseases, where the immune system mistakenly attacks healthy cells, can lead to chronic inflammation.

Additionally, dietary choices high in processed foods, sugars, and unhealthy fats, as well as physical inactivity, can contribute to chronic inflammation. Obesity is also linked to chronic inflammation, and this connection may contribute to cancer risk. Exposure to environmental toxins and pollutants may also trigger chronic inflammation, influencing cancer risk. Hormonal imbalances, particularly those related to estrogen, may also contribute to chronic inflammation and impact breast cancer risk.

To reduce inflammation and potentially prevent cancer, it is important to adopt a healthy lifestyle, including a balanced diet, regular exercise, and stress management. Additionally, including foods with anti-inflammatory properties, such as fruits, vegetables, and omega-3 fatty acids, in the diet may mitigate inflammation.

It is also important to manage and treat underlying conditions that contribute to chronic inflammation, such as infections or autoimmune diseases. Regular health check-ups allow for the monitoring of overall health, including inflammatory markers, and early intervention if necessary.

Finally, recognizing the mind-body connection and incorporating practices such as meditation, yoga, and mindfulness can contribute to overall well-being and may have anti-inflammatory effects. Ongoing research continues to deepen our understanding of the intricate relationship between inflammation and cancer, informing potential preventive strategies.

** Empowering Wellness: Lifestyle Changes to Reduce Inflammation**

Promoting an anti-inflammatory lifestyle is a proactive way to look after your overall health and wellbeing, with potential benefits in reducing the risk of chronic diseases, including cancer. This chapter looks at practical lifestyle changes that individuals can make to create an anti-inflammatory environment within the body.

1. Adopting an Anti-Inflammatory Diet:
   - **Focus on Whole Foods:** Make sure your diet is full of whole, unprocessed foods, such as fruits, vegetables, whole grains, and lean proteins.
   - **Include Omega-3 Fatty Acids:** Incorporate sources of omega-3 fatty acids, like fatty fish (salmon, mackerel), flaxseeds, chia seeds, and walnuts.

2. Limiting Processed Foods:

- **Reduce Added Sugars:** Processed foods often contain high levels of added sugars, which can contribute to inflammation. Cut down on sugary snacks and drinks.
   - **Avoid Trans Fats:** Trans fats, found in some processed and fried foods, are associated with inflammation. Read labels and choose healthier cooking oils.

3. Maintaining a Healthy Weight:
   - **Balance Caloric Intake:** Achieve and maintain a healthy weight through a combination of balanced diet and regular physical activity. Excess body fat is linked to inflammation.

4. Regular Physical Activity:
   - **Do Aerobic Exercise:** Do regular aerobic exercise, such as brisk walking, jogging, cycling, or swimming. Aim for at least 150 minutes per week.
   - **Do Strength Training:** Include strength training exercises to build muscle mass and support overall physical health.

5. Stress Management Techniques:
   - **Practice Mindfulness and Meditation:**
Practice mindfulness and meditation to manage
stress. Chronic stress can contribute to
inflammation, and these techniques promote
relaxation.
   - **Do Yoga:** Incorporate yoga into your
routine, combining physical activity with
stress-reducing benefits.

6. Adequate Sleep:
   - **Prioritize Quality Sleep:** Aim for 7-9
hours of quality sleep per night. Sleep is crucial
for overall health, and insufficient sleep may
contribute to inflammation.

7. Hydration:
   - **Drink Plenty of Water:** Staying hydrated
is essential for overall health. Water helps flush
toxins from the body and supports various
bodily functions.

8. Anti-Inflammatory Herbs and Spices:

- **Use Turmeric and Ginger:** Incorporate anti-inflammatory herbs and spices into your diet, such as turmeric and ginger. These contain compounds with potential anti-inflammatory effects.

9. Limiting Alcohol Consumption:
   - **Moderation is Key:** If you choose to consume alcohol, do so in moderation. Excessive alcohol intake can contribute to inflammation.

10. Smoking Cessation:
   - **Quit Smoking:** Smoking is a significant contributor to inflammation and a risk factor for various diseases. Quitting smoking promotes overall health.

11. Omega-3 Supplements:
   - **Consult with Healthcare Provider:** Consider omega-3 fatty acid supplements after consulting with your healthcare provider. These supplements may have anti-inflammatory properties.

12. Nutrient-Rich Foods:
   - **Get Essential Vitamins and Minerals:** Make sure your diet includes a variety of nutrient-rich foods, providing essential vitamins and minerals that support overall health and may have anti-inflammatory effects.

13. Regular Health Check-ups:
   - **Monitor Inflammatory Markers:** Include regular health check-ups to monitor inflammatory markers. Discuss the results with your healthcare provider for personalized recommendations.

14. Social Connections:
   - **Build Relationships:** Strong social connections and positive relationships contribute to emotional wellbeing, potentially reducing stress and inflammation.

Chapter 10: Nourishing Wellness: The Crucial Role of Nutrition in Breast Health

Nutrition is a key factor in overall health, and its influence on breast health is especially important. This chapter looks at the importance of a balanced diet in promoting breast health and reducing the risk of breast cancer.

1. Essential Nutrients for Breast Health:
  - **Vitamins and Minerals:** Getting enough essential vitamins and minerals, such as vitamin D, vitamin A, vitamin C, and calcium, is essential for overall health and may also benefit breast health.
   - **Antioxidants:** Eating antioxidant-rich foods, like berries, leafy greens, and nuts, helps protect cells from oxidative stress.

2. Maintaining a Healthy Weight:

- **Caloric Balance:** Eating a balanced diet can help with weight management, and maintaining a healthy weight is linked to a lower risk of breast cancer.

3. Whole Foods and Fiber:
  - **Fruits and Vegetables:** Eating plenty of fruits and vegetables provides fiber, vitamins, and antioxidants. Aim for a variety of colors to get a range of nutrients.
  - **Whole Grains:** Incorporate whole grains, such as brown rice, quinoa, and whole wheat, for sustained energy and dietary fiber.

4. Lean Proteins:
  - **Poultry, Fish, and Plant-Based Proteins:** Include lean sources of protein in your diet, such as poultry, fish, legumes, and tofu. Protein is essential for tissue repair and immune function.

5. Omega-3 Fatty Acids:
  - **Fatty Fish, Flaxseeds, and Walnuts:** Omega-3 fatty acids, found in fatty fish,

flaxseeds, and walnuts, have anti-inflammatory properties and may contribute to breast health.

6. Healthy Fats:
   - **Avocado, Nuts, and Olive Oil:** Incorporate healthy fats into your diet, such as those found in avocados, nuts, and olive oil. These fats support overall health and well-being.

7. Hormone-Balancing Foods:
   - **Cruciferous Vegetables:** Broccoli, cauliflower, and Brussels sprouts contain compounds that may help balance hormones and reduce the risk of hormone-related breast cancers.

8. Limiting Processed Foods and Sugars:
   - **Minimize Added Sugars:** Processed foods and added sugars can lead to inflammation and may affect overall health. Limiting their consumption is beneficial.

9. Hydration:

   - **Adequate Water Intake:** Staying hydrated is essential for overall health, including breast health. Water supports various bodily functions and helps flush out toxins.

10. Moderation in Alcohol Consumption:
   - **Moderation is Key:** If you choose to drink alcohol, do so in moderation. Excessive alcohol intake is associated with an increased risk of breast cancer.

11. Bone Health:
   - **Calcium-Rich Foods:** Adequate calcium intake supports bone health. Include dairy products, fortified plant-based milk, and leafy greens in your diet.

12. Prebiotics and Probiotics:
   - **Fermented Foods:** Incorporate prebiotics and probiotics from sources like yogurt, kefir, sauerkraut, and kimchi to support gut health and overall well-being.

13. Individualized Nutrition:

- **Consider Personal Health Factors:**
Customize your diet to your individual health
needs. If you have specific health concerns or
conditions, talk to a healthcare provider or a
registered dietitian for personalized advice.

14. Breastfeeding:
   - **Benefits for Mother and Child:** If
possible, consider breastfeeding. Breastfeeding
has been associated with a reduced risk of breast
cancer and provides numerous health benefits
for both mother and child.

15. Regular Health Check-ups:
   - **Monitor Nutrient Levels:** Regular health
check-ups can include assessments of nutrient
levels. Addressing any deficiencies ensures
optimal support for breast health.

** Nutrient-Rich Allies: Specific Foods for Breast Health**

Certain foods contain nutrients and compounds that have been linked to potential benefits for breast health. This chapter looks at particular foods and nutrients that may contribute to overall wellness and reduce the risk of breast cancer.

Fatty fish, such as salmon, mackerel, and trout, are high in omega-3 fatty acids, which are known for their anti-inflammatory properties. Eating these fish regularly may help support breast health. Berries, like blueberries, strawberries, and raspberries, are packed with antioxidants, which help protect cells from oxidative stress. These compounds may have a positive effect on breast health.

Broccoli, cauliflower, Brussels sprouts, and kale are all cruciferous vegetables that contain sulforaphane, a compound with potential anti-cancer properties. These vegetables may help to balance hormones. Turmeric is rich in curcumin, which has anti-inflammatory and antioxidant properties. Incorporating turmeric into meals may have potential benefits for breast health. Green tea is full of epigallocatechin gallate (EGCG), a catechin with antioxidant properties. Some studies suggest that green tea may have protective effects against breast cancer. Nuts and seeds, such as almonds, walnuts, flaxseeds, and chia seeds, provide omega-3 fatty acids and phytochemicals.

Eating a variety of nuts and seeds can support overall health. Leafy greens, such as spinach, kale, and Swiss chard, are full of essential vitamins and minerals, which can contribute to overall well-being. Garlic contains organosulfur compounds with potential anti-cancer effects. Eating garlic regularly may be associated with a reduced risk of certain cancers. Pomegranates are full of antioxidants, particularly punicalagins and anthocyanins. Some studies suggest potential benefits for breast health. Yogurt, kefir, sauerkraut, and kimchi are all sources of probiotics that support gut health. A healthy gut microbiome is associated with overall well-being. Flaxseeds contain lignans, plant compounds with antioxidant properties.

These may help to balance hormones and potentially reduce the risk of hormone-related cancers. Citrus fruits, such as oranges, grapefruits, and lemons, are high in vitamin C, an antioxidant that supports the immune system and overall health. Extra virgin olive oil is rich in monounsaturated fats and antioxidants. It is a key component of the Mediterranean diet, which has been associated with various health benefits. Soy products, like tofu and edamame, contain isoflavones, which are phytoestrogens. Some studies suggest that soy may have a protective effect against breast cancer. Certain mushrooms, such as shiitake and maitake, contain beta-glucans and antioxidants.

These compounds may contribute to immune support. Tomatoes are rich in lycopene, an antioxidant that may have potential benefits for breast health. Cooking tomatoes enhances the availability of lycopene. Avocado is a source of monounsaturated fats and antioxidants. Eating avocados can support heart health and overall well-being.

Chapter 11: Nature's Potential: Herbal Remedies and Complementary Therapies for Breast Health**

Conventional medical approaches are essential for breast cancer prevention and treatment, but some people also explore complementary therapies, such as herbal remedies. This chapter provides an overview of herbal remedies with potential anti-cancer properties and their role in supporting breast health.

For example,

1. turmeric (Curcuma longa) contains curcumin, an active compound with anti-inflammatory and antioxidant properties that may inhibit cancer cell growth.

2. Green tea (Camellia sinensis) is rich in epigallocatechin gallate (EGCG), a polyphenol with potential anti-cancer effects.

3. Garlic (Allium sativum) contains organosulfur compounds, including allicin, which have demonstrated anti-cancer properties in preclinical studies.

4. Essiac tea is a blend of herbs, including burdock root, sheep sorrel, slippery elm, and Indian rhubarb, that is traditionally used to benefit cancer patients, although scientific evidence is limited.

5. Maitake mushrooms (Grifola frondosa) contain beta-glucans, compounds that may have immunomodulatory effects and contribute to overall health.

6. Cat's claw (Uncaria tomentosa) has anti-inflammatory properties and is believed to have immune-boosting effects.

7. Astragalus (Astragalus membranaceus) is an adaptogenic herb that may enhance the immune system's function.

8. Reishi mushrooms (Ganoderma lucidum) contain polysaccharides and triterpenes, which have demonstrated anti-cancer effects in preclinical studies.

9. Milk thistle (Silybum marianum) is rich in silymarin, an antioxidant that may have hepatoprotective effects.

10. Echinacea (Echinacea purpurea) is known for its immune-modulating effects, although more research is needed to explore its potential in cancer support.

11. Black Cohosh (Actaea racemosa):
  - **Phytoestrogenic Effects:** Black cohosh is known for its phytoestrogenic effects, which may influence hormonal balance. It is studied for its potential role in breast health.

12. Red Clover (Trifolium pratense):
   - **Isoflavones:** Red clover contains isoflavones, plant compounds with estrogen-like properties. It is being explored for its potential in managing symptoms related to hormonal changes.

13. Ginger (Zingiber officinale):
   - **Anti-Inflammatory Properties:** Ginger has anti-inflammatory properties, and some studies suggest it may have anti-cancer effects. It is being investigated for its role in cancer prevention and treatment.

14. Licorice Root (Glycyrrhiza glabra):
   - **Antioxidant and Anti-Inflammatory:** Licorice root has antioxidant and anti-inflammatory properties. It is being studied for its potential role in cancer prevention.

15. Frankincense (Boswellia serrata):
   - **Boswellic Acids:** Frankincense contains boswellic acids, which have demonstrated

anti-inflammatory and anti-cancer effects in preclinical studies.

16. Yarrow (Achillea millefolium):
   - **Anti-Inflammatory and Antioxidant:** Yarrow is known for its anti-inflammatory and antioxidant properties. It is being explored for its potential in supporting overall health.

17. Chamomile (Matricaria chamomilla):
   - **Anti-Inflammatory and Antioxidant:** Chamomile has anti-inflammatory and antioxidant properties. While more research is needed, it is traditionally used for its calming effects.

18. Consultation with Healthcare Provider:
   - **Individualized Approach:** Before incorporating herbal remedies or complementary therapies into breast health management, it is important to consult with a healthcare provider. They can provide guidance tailored to individual health needs.

Holistic Support: The Integral Role of Complementary Therapies in Cancer Care

Cancer care goes beyond traditional medical treatments, taking a holistic approach that considers the physical, emotional, and mental aspects of health. Complementary therapies are an important part of providing holistic support to those dealing with cancer. This chapter looks at the various complementary therapies and their role in cancer care.

Mind-body practices such as meditation and mindfulness can help people manage stress and anxiety, while yoga and tai chi combine gentle movements, breath control, and meditation to promote physical and emotional balance. Acupuncture involves inserting thin needles into specific points on the body to stimulate energy flow and restore balance, and may help with treatment-related symptoms like nausea and pain. Massage therapy can provide relief from treatment-related symptoms, reduce stress, and improve overall quality of life.

Art and music therapy offer creative outlets for self-expression and emotional processing, while nutritional counseling provides personalized guidance on dietary choices to support overall health. Exercise and physical therapy help cancer patients maintain physical function, reduce fatigue, and improve strength. Herbal and dietary supplements may be used under the guidance of healthcare providers to complement conventional cancer care and manage side effects.

Supportive counseling and psychotherapy offer a supportive environment for individuals to navigate the emotional challenges associated with cancer, while energy healing practices such as Reiki and Healing Touch aim to balance and enhance the body's energy flow. Integrative medicine clinics bring together conventional and complementary therapies, and aromatherapy uses essential oils to promote relaxation and alleviate symptoms.

Support groups and peer counseling provide opportunities for individuals facing cancer to share experiences and offer mutual support, while palliative care focuses on alleviating symptoms and improving quality of life. Holistic survivorship programs recognize the importance of ongoing support after treatment, and individualized approaches involve tailoring care to individual preferences, needs, and beliefs.

It is important to have open communication with the healthcare team to ensure safety and alignment with overall treatment goals when considering complementary therapies.

Navigating Safely: Important Considerations and Precautions in Cancer Care

As individuals navigate the various aspects of cancer care, from conventional treatments to complementary therapies, it is essential to approach these choices with knowledge, understanding, and consideration of individual health needs. This chapter will explore important considerations and precautions to ensure a safe and informed journey through cancer care.

1. Open Communication with Healthcare Team:
   - **Transparent Dialogue:** Maintain an open dialogue with your healthcare team. Share your thoughts, worries, and any complementary therapies you are considering.

2. Integration with Conventional Care:
   - **Collaborative Approach:**
Complementary therapies should be seen as

supportive elements to conventional cancer care. They should not replace or interfere with prescribed medical treatments.

3. Individualized Assessments:
  - **Personal Health Status:** Take into account your individual health status, including the type and stage of cancer, overall health, and any existing medical conditions. Complementary therapies should be tailored to your unique needs.

4. Consultation with Healthcare Providers:
  - **Professional Guidance:** Before incorporating any complementary therapy, consult with your healthcare providers. They can provide insights, assess potential interactions, and offer guidance based on your specific health situation.

5. Timing and Treatment Phases:
  - **Consider Treatment Phases:** Some complementary therapies may be more suitable during certain phases of treatment or recovery.

Discuss timing with your healthcare team to align with your treatment plan.

6. Safety of Herbal and Dietary Supplements:
   - **Potential Interactions:** Herbal remedies and dietary supplements can interact with medications. Let your healthcare team know about any supplements you are taking to prevent potential interactions.

7. Potential Side Effects:
   - **Awareness and Monitoring:** Be aware of potential side effects or interactions associated with complementary therapies. Regular monitoring and communication with healthcare providers are essential.

8. Evidence-Based Practices:
   - **Research and Evidence:** Focus on practices supported by scientific evidence. While some complementary therapies may lack extensive research, choose those with a

reasonable level of evidence regarding safety and potential benefits.

9. Professional Practitioners:
   - **Qualified Providers:** If seeking services like acupuncture or massage therapy, choose qualified practitioners with experience in working with cancer patients. Verify their credentials and inquire about their knowledge of your specific condition.

10. Physical Limitations:
   - **Adapt to Physical Needs:** Consider any physical limitations or challenges resulting from cancer or its treatment. Adapt activities or therapies to accommodate your current physical abilities.

11. Emotional and Psychological Impact:
   - **Address Emotional Well-Being:** Complementary therapies, including counseling and support groups, can address emotional and psychological aspects of cancer. Prioritize your mental health and well-being.

12. Financial Considerations:
   - **Budgeting and Insurance:** Some complementary therapies may not be covered by insurance. Consider the financial aspects and explore options that fit your budget.

13. Consistency in Communication:
   - **Updates to Healthcare Team:** Keep your healthcare team informed about any changes in your complementary therapy regimen, ensuring continuity of care and an accurate understanding of your overall health.

14. Holistic Survivorship Planning:
   - **Long-Term Health Considerations:** As you transition into survivorship, engage in holistic survivorship planning. Discuss long-term health considerations, including ongoing monitoring and preventive measures.

15. Informed Decision-Making:
   - **Educated Choices:** Make informed decisions by seeking reliable information,

consulting with healthcare providers, and considering your values and preferences.

Chapter 12: Nurturing the Soul: Emotional and Mental Well-Being in the Face of Breast Cancer

The emotional toll of a breast cancer diagnosis is far-reaching, affecting an individual's overall well-being. This chapter will explore the various facets of emotional and mental health, providing guidance on how to manage the challenges and cultivate resilience throughout the breast cancer journey.

Acknowledging Emotions: It is normal to experience a range of emotions, such as fear, anxiety, sadness, and anger, when faced with a breast cancer diagnosis. It is important to recognize these feelings as valid responses to a life-altering experience.

Open Communication: Sharing your emotions with trusted friends, family members, or a mental health professional can help to lighten the burden and provide comfort and support.

Professional Counseling: Seeking the guidance of a mental health professional, such as a counselor or therapist, can help to navigate complex emotions and develop coping strategies.

Support Groups: Joining a breast cancer support group can offer a sense of community and understanding. Connecting with others who share similar experiences can provide valuable insights and emotional support.

Mindfulness and Meditation: Incorporating mindfulness and meditation practices into your routine can help to manage stress, reduce anxiety, and promote a sense of calm.

Creative Expression: Engaging in creative outlets, such as art, writing, or music, can serve as powerful tools for processing emotions and fostering a sense of empowerment.

Setting Realistic Expectations: It is important to set realistic expectations for yourself and understand that it is okay to experience a range of emotions, and healing is a gradual process.

Self-Compassion: Practicing self-compassion is essential. Treat yourself with the same kindness and understanding that you would offer to a dear friend facing a similar situation.

Resilience Building: Cultivating resilience by identifying and focusing on your strengths can help to guide you through challenges.

Establishing Boundaries: Setting boundaries to protect your emotional well-being is important. Prioritize activities and relationships that contribute positively to your life.

Seeking Spiritual Support: If spirituality is a part of your life, engaging in practices that provide spiritual comfort, such as prayer, meditation, or connecting with a spiritual community, can be beneficial.

Balancing Positivity and Realism: It is important to balance optimism with realism. While maintaining a positive outlook is beneficial, it is also crucial to acknowledge and address difficult emotions.

Holistic Approaches: Exploring holistic approaches that recognize the mind-body connection, such as yoga, tai chi, or acupuncture, can promote overall well-being.

Care for Caregivers: It is important to recognize the emotional impact on caregivers and loved ones. Encourage open communication, and seek support together to navigate the journey as a team.

Professional Guidance for Families: Family counseling can facilitate open communication and understanding among family members. A united support system contributes to emotional well-being.

Survivorship Plans: As you transition into survivorship, work with your healthcare team to create a survivorship plan that addresses emotional and mental well-being in the post-treatment phase.

Breast cancer is not only a physical battle but a deeply emotional one. Taking care of your emotional and mental health is an essential part of the healing journey, fostering resilience and providing a foundation for a life beyond breast cancer.

** Building Bridges of Support: Support Groups, Counseling, and Mental Health Resources**

Navigating the complexities of breast cancer involves more than just medical treatments; it requires a strong network of emotional support and mental health resources. This chapter will explore the invaluable role of support groups, counseling, and mental health resources in providing strength and resilience throughout the breast cancer journey.

Support Groups:
- Community Bonding: Joining a breast cancer support group can create a sense of community where individuals can share their experiences, insights, and emotional support. These groups can be in-person or online, allowing for flexibility based on personal preferences and circumstances.

Professional Counseling:

- Therapeutic Direction: Professional counseling, whether individual or family-based, provides a confidential space to explore emotions, develop coping strategies, and receive guidance from mental health professionals experienced in cancer care.

Oncology Social Workers:
- Comprehensive Support: Oncology social workers specialize in providing support to individuals and families affected by cancer. They offer assistance in navigating practical challenges, emotional support, and access to resources.

Psychotherapy:
- Addressing Mental Health Issues: Psychotherapy, including cognitive-behavioral therapy (CBT) and other therapeutic modalities, can help individuals manage anxiety, depression, and other mental health concerns associated with breast cancer.

Online Forums and Communities:

- Virtual Connections: Online forums and communities provide a virtual space for individuals to connect, share experiences, and seek advice. These platforms offer a sense of community and understanding for those unable to attend in-person support groups.

Peer Counseling Programs:
- Shared Experiences: Peer counseling programs connect individuals with breast cancer survivors who offer support based on their shared experiences. This one-on-one connection provides a unique form of understanding and encouragement.

Cancer Navigators:
- Guiding and Advocating: Cancer navigators are professionals who assist individuals in navigating the complexities of cancer care. They provide guidance, advocacy, and support throughout the treatment process.

Crisis Helplines:

- Immediate Assistance: Crisis helplines, such as helplines for mental health or cancer support, offer immediate assistance for those in crisis or needing someone to talk to.

Community Centers and Wellness Programs:
- Holistic Well-Being: Many community centers and wellness programs offer support services for individuals affected by cancer, including support groups, counseling, and holistic well-being initiatives.

Employee Assistance Programs (EAPs):
- Workplace Support: If applicable, explore Employee Assistance Programs provided by employers. EAPs often offer counseling services and resources to support employees facing personal challenges, including those related to health.

National and Local Organizations:
- Resource Hubs: National and local organizations dedicated to cancer support, such as the American Cancer Society or local cancer

centers, can serve as valuable resource hubs, providing information on support groups, counseling services, and mental health resources.

Mindfulness and Meditation Programs:
- Stress Reduction: Mindfulness and meditation programs, often offered through cancer centers or community organizations, can contribute to stress reduction and emotional well-being.

Holistic Health Centers:
- Integrated Care: Holistic health centers may provide a range of services, including counseling, support groups, and complementary therapies, to address the physical, emotional, and spiritual aspects of well-being.

Public Libraries and Educational Resources:
- Educational Workshops: Public libraries and community centers may host educational workshops on mental health and coping strategies. Attendees can benefit from shared knowledge and mutual support.

Educational Workshops and Webinars:
- Informed Decision-Making: Attend educational workshops and webinars offered by reputable organizations. These resources provide valuable information on mental health, coping strategies, and survivorship.

Survivorship Programs:
- Life After Treatment: Survivorship programs often include mental health components to address the unique challenges individuals face after completing breast cancer treatment.

Financial Assistance Programs:
- Relieving Financial Stress: Financial assistance programs can alleviate the financial burden associated with cancer care, reducing stress and contributing to overall well-being.

Conclusion: Nurturing Health, Embracing Hope

As we wrap up this exploration of the multifaceted world of breast cancer, let's take a moment to reflect on the key information that can help individuals to face their journey with resilience and hope.

We have looked at the causes, types, and stages of breast cancer, the importance of early detection through regular screenings, and the various treatment options, personalized plans, and coping mechanisms. We have also discussed the significance of emotional and mental well-being, the role of support groups, counseling, and mental health resources, and the value of complementary therapies, herbal remedies, and lifestyle changes in a holistic approach to breast health.

It is important to be proactive in our health measures. Regular screenings, a balanced diet, physical activity, and mindfulness can all contribute to overall well-being and help with early detection. Self-awareness and open communication with healthcare providers are essential for proactive health measures. A healthy lifestyle is not just a response to adversity, but a lifelong commitment to well-being.

We must also acknowledge the ongoing research and advancements in the field of breast cancer care. Dedicated researchers and healthcare professionals are continually making new discoveries, developing innovative treatments, and deepening our understanding of the complexities of breast cancer. As we come to the end of this journey, we must recognize the hard work that is driving progress in breast cancer care and the hope it brings for future generations.

Finally, let us remember that each individual's journey is unique, and the path to well-being is multifaceted. Breast cancer does not define us, but rather, it becomes a chapter in a broader narrative of resilience, strength, and hope. As we move forward, let the knowledge we have gained be a source of empowerment, the support we have received be a foundation for resilience, and the hope we have embraced be a guiding light on the path to a healthy, fulfilling life.

May the future be marked by continued progress, heightened awareness, and a shared commitment to a world where breast cancer is not just treatable but preventable. Our journey does not end here; it transforms into a story of survival, resilience, and the indomitable spirit that defines the human experience.

Click For More Instereting books

www.ingramcontent.com/pod-product-compliance
Lightning Source LLC
Chambersburg PA
CBHW070848260726
48661CB00004B/1301